I0429344

DON'T JUST SIT THERE!

FITNESS WALKING FOR ALL AGES

By

CINDY ZAHN

INTRODUCTION

This is book number 4 in my "Don't just sit there!" series.

I am a certified health coach. In all my teachings in this area the one thing that came up time and time again was that you must be involved in some sort of physical activity if you want to stay fit, lose weight, whatever your goal might be. If you come across some diet that says no exercise is need, don't believe it.

When you exercise your heart rate increases, blood flows through your blood vessels at a faster rate. This creates something called nitric oxide. Nitric oxide has many benefits to our body. Some of these are: assisting the immune system at fighting off bacteria and defending against tumors, reduces inflammation and helps with sleep.

Walking is an excellent way to get exercise. It's cheap, it's easy on the body and can be done by all fitness levels. Not only will walking improve your health, but it will give you more energy and lift your spirits.

Table of Contents

Disclaimer

The medical information in this book is not advice and should not be treated as such. The medical information is provided without any representations or warranties, expressed or implied. You must not rely on the information in this book as an alternative to medical advice from your doctor. If you have any specific questions about any medical matter, you should consult your doctor or other professional healthcare provider. If you think that you may be suffering from any medical condition, you should seek immediate medical attention. You should never delay seeking medical advice, disregard medical advice or discontinue medical treatment because of information in this book.

Chapter 1. Walking for fitness for all ages.

Without question, walking is the most common physical activity in the United States. It is easy on the body, it's cheap, it's simple and people of all ages and fitness levels can enjoy a good walk. Whatever your reason for walking, whether it be taking your dog out for a walk around the block, walking to clear your head, or walking as part of a weight-loss program, walking will not only improve your health but give you more energy and lift your spirits.

Walking is so much fun that people of all ages are walking. More of the elderly and senior population are walking than ever before. Walking provides seniors with more energy, fresh air and a great sense of well-being. This in turn adds to their quality of life. Even though everyone should always take safety measures when walking, it's even more important for seniors to follow these important tips.

- Make sure you warm up before starting your walk and cool down when you're finished. You don't have to spend a long time warming up; just long enough to do a few stretches for your legs, arms and back. Walking in place is also a great warm up exercise. Don't try to do too much too soon. Build up your pace, distance and speed gradually.
- Drink plenty of water before during and after your walk, even in cold weather. It is recommended that before you start your walk

you should drink eight ounces of water. Then another eight ounces during the walk and at least that much when you're done.

- Keep to the sidewalks or any paths that may be present. If you are forced to walk near or on the road, make sure you face oncoming traffic that way they will be able to see you as good as you can see them. Avoid walking after dark and avoid dangerous crosswalks or intersections.
- Pay attention to all traffic signals and signs and allow yourself plenty of time to cross the street.
- If you begin feeling dizzy, nauseous or have chest pains, stop immediately and call for help.
- Walk with a friend or as part of a group. It's more fun that way, easier to stay motivated and it's also much safer.
- Stick with your walking and don't give up!

Chapter 2. A Walking Program May Be the Perfect Choice for Losing Weight

Losing weight may be easy for one individual while another may find it a constant struggle. A lot of this might be due to genetics, our metabolism, eating habits or amount of exercise we get. A big reason for people being overweight is from not getting enough exercise. This is very common with individuals that have a job where they are sitting most of the day and then when they go home they end up doing more of the same. I myself can attest to this. I sit all day and when I get home all I want to do is just chill out, relax. I am so tired and drained that the thought of getting out and walking, while I know I should do it, is the last thing I want to do.

Vigorous Exercise Programs Do Not Help

Over time, your muscles and energy system begins to lose efficiency from lack of use. Because your entire body is so out of shape, you often find that an intense exercise program is more than you can handle. While exercises like jogging and running are great for burning calories, they are not meant for those who are not used to consistent exercise. Instead of helping you to lose weight quickly, they force your body to burn carbohydrates, which is going to make you tired much quicker. Many strenuous exercises will not allow your body to exercise at the low level that is required to burn fat. Walking will allow your body to do just that.

Walking Offers You the Perfect Pace

Walking allows you to workout at a pace that's steady, consistent, and works well for just about everybody. These are characteristics that are required to effectively burn fat. Unlike exercises like hockey, baseball or tennis, which has slow periods sometimes followed by great bursts of energy requirements, walking is consistent and constantly in fat-burning mode from the time you start until your walk is finished. A walking program may be the best choice for losing weight and keeping it off.

Exercise that's Fun

Walking will easily become your favorite exercise program, especially if you begin to drop the fat and look really great. But, there are other things that make walking a great choice. It is not only fun but it is something you can do with your family, friends or even your dog. Your dog will love going for a walk with you regularly. And they also make great walking buddies. It's also a great way to socialize with friends. Whether you're walking through the mall, in the park, down the beach or around the block in your neighborhood, walking can easily be the easiest and most effective exercise program you've ever used. You'll find the more you walk, the more you'll want to walk.

CHAPTER 3. STARTING YOUR WALKING FITNESS PROGRAM

Walking is one of the most common types of physical fitness. More people are now walking than ever. Walking provides us with many benefits including great exercise, savings on gas, less highway bottle necking, less pollution and a great way to lose weight. Here are some tips to keep in mind if you are just starting your walking fitness program.

Start off Slow

One of the main errors many novices make with walking is that they try to do too much too soon. They attempt to walk more miles than they are able and are often not dressed properly for the activity and/or the weather. This may result in sore and painful feet and total exhaustion. This may cause discouragement that might lead them from walking again or at least for a while.

When you are just starting, take a short walk for 5 to 10 minutes and come back. You can do this a couple of times a day for the first week. Each week thereafter, add 5 minutes to the walk and keep doing this until you've reached your goal. Few people realize how important it is to maintain good posture and walk tall. Keep your abdominal muscles and buttocks as tight as possible with your head held high and your shoulders back and relaxed.

Take Care of your body

Drink plenty of water before, during and after you have finished walking. Make sure you allow your body a chance to warm up before you start walking. This can be accomplished by doing a few simple stretching exercises. Even if you do not plan on walking far or feel walking is easy, you still need to warm up your muscles and joints to avoid injury and soreness. It's equally important to do some "cooling down" stretches when you're finished walking. The importance of stretching both before and after your walking cannot be overstated and should be a key part of your fitness walking program.

Develop a Pattern

One of the hardest things about starting a walking fitness program is being consistent and doing it every day. When first starting your program you should walk every day, starting slowly and working yourself up to the pace you want. If you have a heart monitor, it can be helpful because you will be able to walk at a speed that will allow you to reach your ideal heart rate. If your reason for walking is the health benefits, then you should walk for 30 minutes each day. A good pace to walk is what is known as a "talking pace". This means although you may have elevated breathing, you can still walk and carry on a normal conversation.

Chapter 4. Being a Smart Walker

Being a Smart Walker

Walking is a lot of fun and a great source of exercise and physical fitness. Here are some tips that can help you to become a smart walker and get the most out of your walks.

Don't forget to warm up

Nothing feels better than getting out for a walk and soaking up the sunshine and warm weather you have waited for all winter long. However, before you strap on your walking shoes and start out, it's very important that you do some warm ups. Eliminating this step can cause some very serious consequences. Sore feet, blisters and bunions are just a few of the discomforts that a good warm up can eliminate. Whether you're a seasoned walker or are just beginning, you still need to give your body a chance to warm up.

There are some easy exercises you can do that will target the muscles that are used the most in walking. These can all be done standing up and they are fairly comfortable.

Two of the exercises involve standing on one foot. In the first exercise, you lift the other foot off the floor and flex your ankle very slowly, doing circles with your toes. Make sure you use the full range of motion and only move your ankle joint, not the leg. Do this exercise 6 times on each leg.

In the second exercise, swing your other leg from the hip. Swing it very loosely front to back in a relaxed motion, making sure your foot is not higher than 12 inches from the floor. Do this 15 to 20 times with each leg.

<u>Cooling Down is Equally Important</u>

As important as it is to warm up before walking, it is just as important to properly cool down afterwards. I know you're tired and stimulated from your walk but you'll be glad you took the time to cool down and your body will thank you.

Stand very still with both feet together. Bend your knees slightly. Let your arms and head hang down loosely towards the floor.   Lean forward from the waist. You will be almost in the position as if you were going to touch your toes but you're not. While you're in that down position, allow your body to stretch and exhale, then stand up very slowly.

With your right hand, grab onto your right toes and pull your foot up and behind you, making sure to keep your right knee facing the ground. Pull your heel towards your buttocks until you feel a slight stretch in your front thigh, shin and hip. While you're doing this, take deep breaths and hold them. Do this on both legs.

Chapter 5. Can I Really Lose Weight By Just Walking?

Losing weight is something we hear about almost every day on the news. We all want to look great. Being overweight can cause many health issues. There are a lot of reasons we want to lose weight. However, dieting is difficult for many people. Whether it's their lifestyle, their desire for good food or just an issue with will power, dieting is not as easy as one thinks. Walking, however, is easy for everyone and is also a great way to lose weight.

<ins>Walking instead of Dieting?</ins>

We have often been told throughout our lives that if we want to lose weight, we have to watch what we eat and/or eat less. Walking gives you the chance to drop extra pounds and get into shape without giving up those great foods you enjoy so much. Don't get me wrong. Watching what we eat and trying to eat healthy is always a good idea. Doing so will not only make it easier to keep our weight down but it will also provide us with a healthier life style. When combined with dieting, walking is probably one of the best weight loss programs available. Not only is walking affordable for any budget but it's fun, it's easy and the benefits are incredible. In addition, when walking with the right techniques and pace, regular walking can help you lose weight even without dieting.

How Can I Lose Weight Without Dieting?

When you're walking and pacing yourself properly, you are telling your muscles what you need them to do with any excess fat or sugars you have in your body. They are, for the time being, to leave the sugars alone (you need some of them for energy) and start burning that excess fat you are carrying around. The more you walk the more fat and calories you burn. You will burn calories when you are walking. Burning calories is how you lose weight. This is especially true when you are burning more calories than you are consuming.

You may be wondering how you can lose weight if you are still consuming a lot of calories. The answer is simple: walk more. Once your body is warmed, walk at a good brisk pace. This will allow your body to burn those calories away. Work yourself up to at least 30 minutes per day of good walking and you will soon see a great improvement in your muscle tone and weight. You'll be amazed at how great you feel and how much energy you have.

Chapter 6. The Easy Way To Count Your Walking Steps

You may or may not have heard about the 10,000 steps a day program where it is said if you walk 10,000 steps, you are walking a distance close to 5 miles. The problem with this program is that the size of the step may vary from person to person. However, for a healthy lifestyle, this is the recommended amount. With the average person, whose step is about 2.5 feet long, it will take more than 2,000 steps to walk a mile. Do you really feel like counting your steps every time you go out walking? What many walkers use to record their steps is a pedometer.

What about the pedometer?

A pedometer is a small device that will tell you how far you have walked. It is also known as a step counter. This useful device makes it very easy for walkers to know when they have reached their target goal. Because its step count is based on the swing of the person's hips, the actual mileage may vary with different individuals of different size. However, it's still regarded as an excellent tool for walkers.

Pedometers are great for providing walkers with motivation. The 10,000 steps guideline is a recommended amount that equals around 5 miles. If an individual leads a sedentary lifestyle, they may only walk 1,000 to 2,000 steps each day. They know they have to increase their steps. The pedometer makes it easy for them to see the number of steps taken each day. They can improve upon this by increasing their number of steps every day till they reach the recommended 10,00 steps.

Increasing your Steps

Increasing your steps to the recommended amount is easier than you may think. Begin to increase it a little each day. An increase of 500 steps each day is a great way to get up to 10,000 per day. As soon as you get up in the morning, place the pedometer on your body and let it start calculating. I personally like to attach my pedometer on my shoe. Some people will attach it to a pocket, or at the waist band of the pants. You can place it where ever it works for you. When first starting out with your pedometer, check it occasionally to make sure it is working properly. At the end of an "average" day, you will know exactly where you stand and what you need to do for improvement. Every day may be different for you. Some days you may be more active than others.

You may find that wearing your pedometer will also make you more motivated to walk more. At the end of a week, you will know how much improvement is needed.

Some things you can do to improve the number of steps you take include:

- Walking your dog
- Taking a walk with a family member or friend

- Taking the stairs in buildings instead of the elevator
- Park farther away from the store so you have to walk more
- Walk to the store if possible
- Get off the couch to change the channel instead of using the remote control

CHAPTER 7. STAYING HYDRATED WHILE WALKING

The old saying of not needing to drink unless you're thirsty does still hold true when you're walking as it's extremely important for your body that you keep it replenished with fluids. When you're walking, you're sweating and, therefore, getting rid of a lot of the fluids in your body. It's important for your health that you refill your body with fluids. This will also make it easier for you to continue walking comfortably.

What kind of fluids should you drink?

The kind of fluids that you should drink when walking will have a lot to do with the kind of walking as well as the duration. Sports drinks are recommended if you're planning on walking for 30 minutes or more, such as a marathon or walkathon. Sports drinks have electrolytes and carbohydrates that will not only provide your body with energy but will also help your body to absorb water quicker.

Some walkers try to dilute the sports drinks or eliminate them altogether to avoid consuming the calories. Diluting them will only decrease the benefits of the drink. It's important for your body that you drink sports drinks that have carbohydrates. You may choose a drink that's low calorie but will still replace the salt you're losing when you walk. Many specialists recommend that you drink whatever beverage you enjoy the most as long as you're drinking something.

A lot of bikers select plain cold water. The best way to decide if you should drink is if you are thirsty. Your body will not lie to you.

How much should you drink?

It can be just as hazardous to drink too much as it can be to not drink enough. If you don't drink enough, you can become dehydrated. If you drink too much, you can get hyponatremia (low blood salt level and fluid overload). Weigh yourself both before and after you begin walking. A rule of thumb is that you should not have a weight loss or gain of more than 2%. If you do, it is an indication that you've been drinking either too much or too little.

A good rule of thumb for walkers is one cup of water for every mile walked. Your weight will also determine the amount. Obviously, the slower you walk, the less water you will need because you won't be losing it as fast. All things said, let your body do a lot of the deciding for you.

CHAPTER 8. IMPROVING YOUR BLOOD PRESSURE THROUGH WALKING

Walking is an activity that more and more people are choosing and they are choosing it for a many reasons. Not only is it relaxing, great for the body and fun, but it also has many health benefits. Latest studies indicate that people that spend more time walking have less problems with high blood pressure.

A study that was in the Journal of Hypertension says that even taking a short but brisk walk for 10 minutes can lower your blood pressure for up to 11 hours. Taking a 45-minute walk will keep the blood pressure down for seven hours. Imagine the great impact walking would have on your blood pressure if you took to 45 minute walks per day.

Get Rid of High Blood Pressure the Easy Way

Many people suffer from prehypertension, which is elevated blood pressure that usually turns into high blood pressure. High blood pressure affects millions of people in America today. This can put them at risk of heart disease, stroke, kidney failure and more. The best treatment for prehypertension is following a good diet and getting sufficient exercise. Walking is a great form of exercise for prehypertension.

Individuals that were part of an independent study walked constantly on a treadmill for 40 minutes on day one. The next day they walked for 10 minutes each four different times over a period of 3.5 hours. The result of this walking was their systolic blood pressure dropping approximately 5.5 mmHg, which is enough of a drop to make a significant difference in their being at risk of heart disease and stroke. The moral of the story is even a few short walks each day can make a difference.

Fit it into Your Schedule

Walking is an activity that is very pleasurable for most people, even those that do not consider themselves as active. The main reason why most people do not get enough walking is their schedule. They don't feel they have time to take long walks. The good news is that a short 10-minute walk once or twice a day can make a big difference in their blood pressure. Think about walking to your favorite restaurant on your lunch hour. The ten minutes you will spend walking is ten minutes you would have used getting to your car and then parking it by the restaurant. And you will feel so much better.

So, whether you can fit long walks into your schedule or only have time for a couple short walks, make the most of them. Grab your water bottle, put the leash on your dog and away you go towards lower and healthier blood pressure.

Chapter 9. Having The Right Walking Gear

Walking is not only a free form of physical fitness but is also one of the easiest fitness activities. You get the urge to go for a walk to get a little exercise and all you do is put on your walking shoes and away you go. However, many people become more dedicated in their walking and have a desire to get special clothing and accessories. Although you don't really need all these accessories, many people enjoy the idea of having a great collection of walking accessories, especially if they're planning on participating in a walking or other fitness activity. Here are some of the essentials for walking.

- Shoes are the most important of your accessories and should be a good pair of shoes designated for walking. There should be plenty of room in the toe area, should have a flexible sole and a comfortable fit.

- Socks are almost as important as your shoes. When you're trying on shoes to buy, make sure you wear the same type of socks you'll be wearing when you're walking so you get a proper fit. Rather than wearing an all-cotton sock, you may want to consider getting socks made of cool max as they'll keep your feet dryer and more comfortable.

- Clothing should be whatever you're comfortable wearing. Fabrics that have wicking characteristics work best because they repel moisture and will keep you dry. When you are planning on walking, make sure you dress for the weather and wear layers of clothing because it's easier to remove excess clothing.

- Sunglasses and a hat are good things to have as well. My eyes are very sensitive to bright sunlight, so sunglasses are a must. And wearing a hat helps protect your head, hair, eyes, neck and face from harmful sun rays. If you are a senior citizen, a hat should be something that you should use regularly. Since you are more prone to dizziness and fatigue, you need more protection.
This is most important during the summer when the sun is strong. Seniors also have much less hair on their head so they do not have the necessary protection from harmful sun rays.

- Water is very important when you're walking so make sure to drink plenty of water both before you begin walking and when you're done. If you're going to be walking for a long time, make sure you drink some water every 20 minutes. You might want to purchase a hydration belt. This is something that you can attach around your waist. They come in various styles from a single water bottle carrier to multiple water bottles. The water bottle(s) are included. Some have pouches built in where you can put things such as cash, your phone, etc. When I go out and walk in the summertime and do about 5 miles, I wear a hydration belt that has two water bottles.

- Many walkers bring along a pedometer so they can keep track of the miles they're walking. Some of the newer models of pedometers have special features that calculate your speed, distance and even the number of calories you're burning.

- Heart rate monitors are also handy devices used by many walkers. They're great to have in that they can tell you how fast your heart is pumping. They can be easily worn around your chest with a belt or in as a wristwatch display.

Walking when the weather gets cold

I live in the northeast. I have a very low tolerance for cold. I enjoy walking outside. So when the weather starts turning cold, I tend to put a halt to my regular walking routine. When I feel up to it, I will go to the local mall and walk, but not as much as I know I should. I guess I could join a gym again.

If you choose to walk during the cold winter months, having warm apparel is imperative, unless you are one of those lucky people who isn't bothered by the cold as much as I. If you are one of those, then go for it.

CHAPTER 10. THE IMPORTANCE OF WALKING

Many Benefits of Walking

Walking has become a very real and enjoyable way of life. Not only is it fun and great exercise but it also has many other benefits. Walking is a great means of transportation. It reduces congestion on the highways, reduces pollution brought on by the millions of cars and trucks on the road and also helps to preserve our non-renewable resources by eliminating the amount of gasoline that has to be used in the millions of vehicles on our highways and roads. And, let's not forget about the high cost of gas, which seems to be increasing every time we turn around. Walking is free and those that choose to walk instead of driving in the car are saving a lot on bus fares, gasoline and other forms of public transportation.

Beneficial to both men and women

We have been told the many benefits that walking provides for us as a whole, but we often don't think about the many health benefits it provides to us on an individual basis. One example is how walking can help prevent many health problems from developing in men or can even resolve the health problems.

Walking will improve your metabolism by providing you with a good digestive system as well as increasing your appetite. All of these things will contribute towards overall better health. Walking is very beneficial for both men and women in reducing stress. Seldom will a person go walking and think about their problems as walking has a way of clearing the head. It is not known whether it's the fresh air that helps to clear the mind or the way your arms and legs move that take stress from both the mind and body, but walking definitely does its magic for all.

Addition Benefits of Walking

Other benefits of walking include:

- Walking helps you to digest your food better. This is particularly beneficial for those that tend to have a diet that consists of heavy and/or fried foods. Walking on a regular basis helps to digest these foods quicker and easier.
- Walking can help you maintain your weight. Those that work long hours on jobs that are sedentary tend to gain extra pounds. Walking regularly can keep this in check.
- Walking provides some great leisure time as well as giving time to socialize with friends. Our busy lives tend to leave us with little time for catching up with friends, but walking will give you back that chance.
- Those who walk regularly claim they feel more energetic, happier and are able to work and move at a much faster pace and still remain healthy.

CHAPTER 11. SETTING YOUR GOALS FOR WALKING

We all know how important walking is for exercise. Not enough people spend time walking. If your life is so busy that you don't manage to fit walking into your schedule, try to set aside one or more days of the week when you get out and walk. You will not only feel better physically but you'll also feel better emotionally. Before you begin your weekly walking, make sure you know what you have planned and try to stick with it. Too many people try to start out with big plans of walking a great distance and are only setting themselves up for failure. I have a full-time day job where I sit most of the day. I find it difficult to get out and walk during the week. But I do get out every Saturday and Sunday, weather permitting, and do at least five miles. Some mornings I really don't feel like it, but I do it anyhow for two reasons. One, if I don't do it, I will be beating myself up all day about it. And number 2, once I get out there and get going, I'm glad I did. I'm thinking that now being that my work hours are not so long, I might be able to fit in a quick walk around the block during the week. We'll see.

Starting off Slow is Vital

The most important thing is to start off slow. If you have been walking for a while, you can continue doing what you've been doing all along. If you're new to walking or are getting back to it after a long break, start off slow. Irrespective of how much pressure you are getting from co-workers about that 5K walkathon this weekend, you are not ready for that yet. When you first begin walking, don't walk any more than what makes you comfortable.

When you start to feel discomfort, it's time to turn around and go home. Don't wait until you're already uncomfortable. Remember, that you still have to walk back home. Even if your first walk is only ten minutes, walk at a pace and duration that is right for you. If you are walking for exercise, make sure you use a proper technique, which means good body movements and, more importantly, good posture.

Setting Goals

Walking has many good health benefits, especially for your heart. You may want to measure the intensity of your walking by keeping track of your heart rate. Many dedicated walkers wear an electronic device that keeps track of it for them. Even if you're only walking for short distances, you're still doing your body good. Try to set goals for yourself where you increase your intensity a little each day as well as the distance or time you spend walking.

A nifty thing to have, if you can afford one, is a fitness band or a sports watch. Most of these things provide an electronic tracking program where all you need to do is plug it into your computer and it downloads and saves the data from your walk. I have used both and wouldn't want to walk without one.

The important thing with goals is to be realistic. Don't set a goal so high that you're only setting yourself up for failure. But, set some sort of goal that you know is realistic and work towards meeting that goal. Walking is wonderful, but if you start walking and then stop for a while and start up again, you are going to have to start slow every time you start up again.   So, decide what a good goal is for you, start walking and have fun! If you happen to have a dog, they'll love joining you.

Chapter 12. The Good News about Walking

Why Walking is so great

Almost everyone enjoys walking. I mean, what's not to like about it? It's very easy to do, it's free (how many things can you actually say that about?), and it's great for the body. Putting it simply, walking is good for you. It's good for everyone. It's a great aerobic exercise and is even good for people that have recently had surgery.

Years ago, it was recommended that patients have weeks of bed rest after surgery. Today, however, physicians recommend that patients get up and start walking a day or two after surgery and walk every day for a fast recovery. Walking helps to reduce your chance of blood clots, helps to keep the heart pumping and also helps you to have less body fat. You always hear some of the most common benefits of walking but are not always aware of just how great walking is for us.

Walking for better circulation

Walking provides your body with better circulation by increasing your heart rate, strengthening your heart, lowering your blood pressure and preventing heart disease in general. Women walking two miles a day can lower their blood pressure by 11 points over a period of six months. A 30-minute daily walk can also reduce women's risk of stroke by 20 percent.

Walking helps bones and joints

Walking helps make the bones and joints stronger and less likely to become fractured. Postmenopausal women will reduce their risk of hip fractures by 40 percent by walking just 30 minutes every day. In addition to supporting our joints, walking also tones up the supporting muscles, particularly the abdominal, leg and arm muscles. Patients with osteoporosis will have less bone mass loss when walking is part of their daily routine. This is because walking helps to provide our joint cartilages with oxygen and other important nutrients by keeping them supplied with the fluids they need to keep moving. Another important factor resulting from this is the reduction of arthritic pain.

Walking may extend your life

There is just no two ways about it. Walking is great for every part of your body. By adding walking to your daily routine, your weight loss program or to your exercise regime, you will be adding years to your life. Where else can you find a free activity that can add years to your life and still be so much fun?

CHAPTER 13. DO I NEED DIFFERENT SOCKS AND SHOES FOR WALKING?

Walking is a very popular form of exercise, whether you're doing it for enjoyment, to spend time with a loved one or friend, to walk your dog or as part of a physical fitness program. Few people realize the importance of wearing the right shoes and socks. While it may be true that years ago people did not have the variety of walking and running shoes we now see on the market, it is also true that they suffered a lot from sore feet.

Whether you're just going to be in a long walkathon or you're planning on walking regularly for exercise, make sure you wear the correct shoe and socks. Here are some tips on the kind of shoes and socks you'll want to wear when you're out walking.

<u>Well cushioned shoes</u>

It has been said that your feet can take 2000 tons of weight every day and if this is true, don't they deserve some cushioning? You may think that you can walk in any kind of shoe but you'll be able to go a lot further and in much more comfort if you're wearing the right kind of shoe. Choose a shoe that is made for walking and you'll be able to go longer and better. The best time of day to try on shoes is late in the day because feet often swell as the day goes on.

Wear the same kind of socks you'll be wearing when you buy the shoes so you get the best possible fit.

Make sure they seem flexible and will easily support your weight. Make sure the shoe has enough room in the toe-box for you to easily move and wiggle your toes. The heels should be firm. Try them on and walk around in the store a little bit with them on. If they're not comfortable in the store, they will NOT be comfortable when you're walking. I was told by an associate in a running store that you should buy shoes that are a size bigger than you normally wear. This is because when walking your feet will swell up. Also make sure you buy the right shoe for your arch type. If possible, it's best to buy your shoes at a store where they have salespeople who are knowledge about what you want to purchase.

Socks make a difference

Your socks should be more than just a fashion statement to match your outfit. You should be willing to take as good care of your feet as they take care of you. Socks have two purposes. They protect your feet from getting injured and they also "wick away" perspiration and keep your feet dry and protect the shoe. Without socks, your perspiration can easily damage the lining of the shoe and make your shoes become very uncomfortable. Once this happens, your feet may get painful blisters or corns.

Choose socks that will provide cushioning for your feet as well as wick away perspiration. Cotton socks will absorb the moisture and feel good but cotton/synthetic blends will help the moisture to evaporate. Socks with padded toes and heels will give your feet a great feeling. If your socks feel moist, change them. Your feet will never stop thanking you for such good care.

Chapter 14. Walking at Charity Events

I don't know too many things that will give people more motivation to walk than knowing their doing it either for their favorite charity or for a charity that affects a loved one. Walking is very popular today and more people than ever are choosing it as their method of exercise and weight control.

What does walking for charities mean?

Walking for charities means just what the phrase indicates. You're walking for a specific charity to raise money. When you choose a specific charity to raise money for by walking, you approach friends and family members and ask them if they're willing to pledge you in that charity. A person may make a flat donation of a certain dollar amount or they may choose to pledge you so much per mile. At the end of the "walkathon", you let them know how many miles you've walked and they give you the money. For instance, if someone pledged you 50 cents a mile and you walked 10 miles, they'd give you 5 dollars, which would go to your favorite charity.

Why walk for charity?

Walking for charities is a great way to get in some good exercise, meet and socialize with many others and raise money to help the charity. Some of the most common charities are to help fight cancer, breast cancer, cystic fibrosis, heart disease and more. Every year more charities are started by people that have a great heart and are willing to donate their time to getting these events going. Walking for charities allows you to be able to make a contribution to any of these great causes while still getting in your favorite exercise. Often as an incentive, the top finishers of the walkathon will be given a prize that's been donated.

Why getting in shape for walk with charities is important?

The idea of becoming part of a charity walk sounds great. You will be with friends, family members or co-workers, you will be getting exercise and you will be helping a worthy cause. However, if you're not in shape for walking, you better get in shape fast. If you are collecting pledges, you need to be in good shape so that you can walk a nice distance so you can collect as much as possible for the charity.

If you are out of shape and the charity walk is "right around the corner", don't do it. You do not want to injure yourself. Charity walks tend to be long and if you are not in shape, you may still try to push yourself to keep up with others and end up in a lot of pain. If there is time, start walking and getting in shape.

CHAPTER 15. WHY YOU SHOULD WALK MORE

Walking is an excellent way to become more physically active. Walking is free, it's fun and the benefits are excellent. Few people fully realize the importance walking can play in their lives. In fact, of all the ways we can be physically active, walking is by far the easiest.

When your exercise schedule includes walking, there are no worries. You can walk any time regardless of where you may be. Walking is also one of the cheapest forms of exercise. The only requirement is a good pair of shoes.

Here are some of the other reasons why we should all make an effort to spend more time walking:

- Walking will leave you feeling energetic and when you have more energy, you just naturally feel better about yourself and everything around you.
- Walking is very relaxing and is a great way to relieve stress. Who doesn't have stress they would like to get rid of?
- Walking helps to put more tone into your muscles and make your muscles and bones stronger.
- Walking will improve your stamina and provide you with overall better physical fitness.
- Walking more will help to lower your risk of chronic diseases such as coronary heart

disease, respiratory problems, diabetes and more.

- Walking will also give you a chance to socialize with your family and friends.

There are many reasons why we should all spend more time walking, and the health benefits is only just the beginning of what it will do for you. As you already know, walking is free so therefore, think of all the money you can save by walking on the many short trips you take every day. The wear and tear you will save on your vehicle should be enough to make you think more seriously about walking instead of driving every chance you get.

If you're the type of person that enjoys doing things with others, ask some of your friends or family members if they would like to join you on for a walk. You may be surprised to find out they have exactly the same feeling about walking alone as you and would love the opportunity to walk with you.

CHAPTER 16. WALKING IS GREAT FOR THE PSYCHE

Walking is one of the most popular pastimes for physical fitness. You've heard all the hype about how good it is for weight loss, firming up your body, and improving your total health. All these things are true. Walking is excellent for your body. But did you know it's also good for the minds as well? Research has found that physical activity such as walking will really help you hone up on your mental skills as well.

Walking will keep Your Brain Bright

If you have ever heard someone say they were going for a walk to clear their head, then you know how true it really is about walking being great for improving the mind. Walking will give you a mental boost that you just can't get anywhere else with so little effort, Walking improves your ability to focus, making it easier to solve problems and make decisions. Just a 15-minute walk will do wonders towards increasing your brain power. The great thing about walking and the benefits for your brain power is that it doesn't suddenly disappear when you stop walking.

Let Walking Perk You Up

Walking has more benefits than most people are even aware of. If you are having a bad day, a walk really can perk your spirits up and make you feel better. Now, it won't make your problems disappear, but it will allow you to clear your head so you can think happier thoughts and improved your mood in general. When you're under stress, walking is a great way to ease away some of your problems.

You may be asking how is that possible? Well, walking releases adrenaline into your body. Adrenaline is a hormone that plays a major role in our nervous system and will give your mood a big boost. Walking also helps the release of endorphins into your body, which not only relieves pain but leaves your entire body with a sense of peacefulness and well-being. You don't need to take a real long walk for your brain to benefit from this physical activity. Several short walks will help you as well.

Walking is great for meditating

Many people that walk on a regular basis use it as a time for thinking, meditating or even praying. They may choose to walk alone so they can think clearly without any disturbances. Walking also will make your body tired so you'll sleep better at night. When you get a good night's sleep, your mind is sharper and more alert. So, start walking and buff your brain regularly.

CHAPTER 17. WALKING, THE ALL AMERICAN PAST TIME

The world as a whole is more health conscious than ever. This is mostly because of all we are exposed to on a daily basis from the news, and other venues, about physical fitness and healthy eating leading to longer, healthier lives.

Walking vs. Exercise Facilities

The world is filled with facilities to fulfill our need and desire for exercise. Hardly a town can be found that doesn't have a public gym, fitness center or weight loss program. Unfortunately, many people can't afford the membership fees that are involved in joining these facilities or can't seem to fit them into their already busy lives. After working all day, driving the kids to their endless amount of activities, who has time to drive and then spend hours at a fitness center? After all, there are only so many hours in the day.

Walking is something that can be easily fit into your daily life, without ever having to leave your yard. While you are cooking dinner, you can easily take a quick walk around the block. Employees are also choosing to walk to their favorite restaurant on their lunch hour, when possible, rather than fighting the busy traffic. Walking is definitely becoming America's favorite past time. Not only is walking great exercise but with the right person it can be a lot of fun. Walking allows you the chance to catch up with your friends and family members and keep up with what's going on in their lives. The best thing about walking is that with all the other many benefits it provides, it's also free. You cannot use the excuse that you cannot afford it. Walking comes with a price that cannot be beat.

What's So Great About Walking?

Sometimes we want to be around others and catch up on the latest news or just chat with them while we exercise but sometimes we just want to be alone with time to think and reflect. Walking allows you that option because you can choose whether you walk alone or with a friend or family member.

Walking also gives you the chance to get some fresh air. Exercise is so important for our overall health and walking is great therapy for the heart. It keeps the blood circulating better and improves the pumping of the heart. People with breathing difficulties also benefit greatly from walking outdoors, absorbing fresh air and sunshine. Walking is great for everyone.

Chapter 18. Walk with the dog.

Walking and exercise in general are playing a larger part in our lives than ever before. With all the new health-related news regarding the importance of good physical fitness for longevity, more people are fitting exercising in their lives. Walking is still the most popular form of exercise.

Walking is the one type of exercise that we are all able to fit into our busy schedules, even if it is just walking those few extra blocks to the store as opposed to taking the car. Walking is fun, it's therapeutic and it's extremely good for our health, particularly our heart.

Man's Best Friend

Another thing that is playing a much larger part in our daily lives is our family dog. Dogs may have been around since the beginning of time, but their role in the family has changed. Years ago, the family dog was often kept outdoors and utilized as a watchdog, farm dog or family pet, never to leave the home. We knew the role of our family dog and the dog knew its role and its duties.

Today, however, dogs are seen everywhere. They are going with their families on vacation. They are seen on the beach, on the sidewalk and any other place that happens to be pet friendly. We are also seeing more pet friendly businesses with the increasing time families are spending with their faithful friend. Many rest stops along the highway can now be seen with a dog runs.

<u>Physical Fitness for Both</u>

Dogs love walking. In fact, there are few things a dog will look forward to more than a nice long walk with its owner. The great thing about walking your dog is that you are providing both of you with not only some great bonding time but also exercise that will promote good health for both. Many people don't realize this, but dogs need exercise just like humans, particularly indoor dogs that seem to spend a large majority of their time eating and sleeping. Can you imagine if all we did was eat and sleep?

If you are looking for a fun way to get some exercise from walking, why not consider taking your dog for a daily walk? You will have a great time and you will be giving your four legged friend a daily treat they will look forward to almost as much as their dog biscuit.

CHAPTER 19. WALKING TO GET IN SHAPE

If you are like a large percentage of the population, winter has been far too long as far as being indoors and idle. I know there are many activities you can do in the winter. And you can also exercise indoors. However, I'm not a winter person myself and while I try to exercise regularly, my plans don't always come to fruition. Now that spring is almost here, however, it is time to put on the walking shoes, get outdoors and get some good old fashioned walking in.

Start Slow

If you have been lazier than you care to admit, there are some steps you may want to take before you start out walking to avoid any possible soreness and discomfort. Even though we hate admitting how out of shape we really are, we tend to find out the hard way with sore and aching muscles the next day! The old saying, "no pain, no gain", really should not apply when it comes to exercise. Usually once your body reaches the point where it's sore, you have done too much too soon and probably didn't do your body any good either.

Proper Clothing

Wear clothing that is loose fitting and in layers so you can always remove some if you become hot. I have found that when layering, if you are layering a short sleeved and long sleeved top together, if you are planning on removing one once you warm up, wear the short sleeved top underneath the long sleeved one. It took me a while before I realized this. I would go out with the short sleeved top over the long sleeved. After a short while I would start getting warm, but there was no way I could remove the one shirt without taking off the other. And believe me, I did experience a few times where I almost just went behind a tree or a building to make the change. If it is cold outside, layers of clothing will keep you warmer than one heavy bulky item of clothing. If you are walking at night, wear reflective tape or bright colors.

Good Walking Shoes

As stated previously, make sure you have some comfortable walking shoes. Shoes really do make a difference. When you are walking, you should have good walking shoes. Your feet will be doing all the work for you so treat them right and protect them.

Warm Up

Regardless of how good of shape you claim to be in, don't ever underestimate the importance of warming up before you begin walking. Start off walking really slow for a few minutes just to get your muscles warmed up. Walking in place will help as well. After you feel you have warmed up, do a few muscle stretches for your calves, hamstrings and quadriceps. Once you feel warm and limber, you are ready to go.

Chapter 20. Walking to Lose Weight

People are becoming more health conscious every day and are adding exercise into their daily lives as part of goal for healthier living. Many more options are available to us today for exercise and physical fitness including gyms, workout centers, fitness programs, weight loss programs and more. With so many more options available it may come as a surprise that many people are still choosing to walk as a way to stay fit and/or lose weight. Walking is fun, it's easy and it's something you can do with a friend or even your dog. Not only are you getting in some good exercise but you're giving your dog a real treat. Dog walking is becoming especially popular with the world becoming more pet friendly.

Walking as Part of a Weight Loss Program

Although most people walk to get into shape or stay in shape, many are using walking as part of a weight loss program. Can you lose weight by just by walking without dieting? Yes, with the right kind and amount of walking, you can and will lose weight. Millions of people are successfully losing weight from their dedication to walking. In fact, walking every day at a moderate pace for 30 to 60 minutes will not only help your body to burn up fat that's stored in your body but will also speed up your metabolism, both which will result in weight loss. Walking regularly at a moderate pace will burn fat and calories.

What Speed Should I Walk To Lose Weight?

Before you begin a long walk at a fast pace, it's important that you start off slow. Begin a slow easy walk for 5 to 10 minutes just to let your muscles know what you are doing. They will get the hint that they're not supposed to burn up available sugar in your body but that instead they need to call on the fat reserves sitting in your body. Get the picture yet? If you start off walking fast, your muscles will burn your sugars instead, which will result more in your becoming fatigued than in actual weight loss.

The speed of walk that's best for weight loss is described as a determined pace, like someone with a purpose in mind. If you're keeping track of your heart rate, it should be 60 to 70 percent of your maximum heart rate and your breathing should allow you to carry on a full conversation while walking. Although it may take a few days, work yourself up to a goal of 30 minutes per walk. Once you've reached that point, do this on a regular basis and as often as possible and you'll soon notice the weight loss.

CHAPTER 21. WALKING YOUR WAY TO GOOD HEALTH

There is so much more to walking than most people realize. While it's a great form of exercise, a method of transportation and a lot of fun, walking also provides our body with many health benefits. In addition to the many health benefits it provides for us, it also reduces our risk of getting many diseases. We hear constantly about some new herb or supplement on the market that will prevent many diseases, but unlike these aids, walking will not cause any side effects.

Weight management is a major reason why many people enjoy walking regularly. Physical fitness is the main thing on the minds of many people today. While they may have trouble dieting, they find that walking is great for not just burning fat and calories but also for keeping them off. Keeping your weight at a healthy amount will decrease your chances of heart disease, type 2 diabetes, cancer, stroke, osteoarthritis, sleep apnea and more.

High blood pressure is a concern for many people, but not as much a concern for those who walk regularly. Physical activity like walking makes the heart stronger so it will pump more blood with a lot less effort or stress on the arteries. Many physicians say that staying in good physical condition is every bit as effective as medication for maintaining good blood pressure levels.

Good cholesterol is something that many people strive for and often fail to achieve without a doctor's care or special diet. Walking will help reduce your low-density lipoproteins (AKA bad cholesterol), which is a leading cause of heart attacks because of the plaque buildup they cause on the walls of your arteries.

Lower your chance of heart attack and stroke by walking regularly. Brisk walking at least three hours each week can low your chances of heart disease by up to 40 percent. All you need to do is walk for a half hour each day. This same walking, increased to an hour a day will cut your chances of a stroke in half.

Gallstone surgery can possibly be eliminated with regular walking every day. If not eliminated, it can lessen your chances of requiring gallbladder surgery by up to 30 percent. Breast cancer and diabetes are two very serious diseases that might be hindered by the use of regular exercise like walking.

These are a few of the many benefits of regular walking. There are far too many ways to mention how walking can help:

- Stronger bones, muscles and joints

- Prevents depression
- Prevents constipation, colon cancer, impotence and osteoporosis
- Lower stress levels
- Improves your sleep
- Relieves arthritis and arthritic pain
- Improves your entire disposition

Chapter 22. Walking Your Way to the Ideal Weight

The benefits of walking are so extraordinary that it would take too long to address each and every one of them. People walk for many reasons. Some work for the fun of it and it surely is a lot of fun. Others walk for the many health benefits. Still others choose to walk as their method of transportation to save on gas and provide them with exercise they may not otherwise get.

Walking is the best

Walking is truly one of the best exercises for maintaining weight and is also great for losing weight. Many people trying to lose weight often times have trouble staying with the diet or find that some of the exercises they are doing are not giving any results or not giving them as quickly as they would like.

It takes time to lose fat permanently, even with exercise and dieting. It is important that you start off with an exercise that will burn fat while, at the same time, bring your fitness to a higher level to burn calories and speed up your weight loss. The perfect exercise for this is walking. By starting off slowly and pacing yourself, you will slowly but surely see results that you'll love.

Slow but Steady Weight Loss

Although walking will not promise that you will lose a lot of weight in a short amount of time, you will lose weight with walking and it will be a permanent weight loss. Some very obvious benefits walking provides you include decrease in health risks, increase in good health and fitness, more energy and higher percentage of body fat burned than any other exercise.

Walking will provide you with a well-toned body while it continues to help your burn the fat and calories. A couple of factors that also make walking so popular are that it is a fun pastime with friends, it's free, it's easy and it doesn't require the use of expensive equipment.

If you have been exercising regularly and are not satisfied with the results, you may wish to try walking either as an alternate to your exercise or as part of your routine. You'll love the way you feel about walking and how much better it will make you feel.

Chapter 23. Ways To Stay Motivated With Your Walking Program

Deciding to put yourself on a walking program is the first step towards getting in better shape and adding years to your life. There are many health benefits that can be gained from walking not to mention all the pleasure you will get from being outdoors. Unfortunately, many people start off with good intentions of walking regularly but either get sidetracked or quickly lose their motivation. Here are some tips on how to stay motivated with your walking program.

<u>Set goals for yourself</u>

As with your walking, start off with small goals that are realistic and achievable. If your goals are too "out of reach", it will be very easy to get discouraged and quit. This is especially true if you haven't been exercising in a while. If you are just starting out, a good goal may be to go on a couple five minute walks per day. Once that becomes easy, you can increase it up to 15 to 20 minutes each time. If you try to do too much too soon, you may end up with pain or an injury, which is a major reason why many people quit walking. The key is to start slow and work yourself up to your final goal.

Vary your walking

Don't walk the same route every time or you'll quickly become bored. The more interesting your walk, the longer you'll want to be walking. Even though your walking program may be your main source of exercise, you can still mix it up with other activities such as biking, soccer with your kids, jumping rope or any number of physical activities that you're familiar with.

Make it fun

The more fun you can make your walking program, the more likely you'll be to stick with it. If there's something about your workouts that you're not comfortable with, try something different. Ask a friend or family member to walk with you. It's always more fun when you're spending time with good company that you enjoy.

I like to have my iPod with me when I walk. The music on it gets me moving and keeps me going. Sometimes I will put a podcast or an audible book on if I need a change of pace.

Make your walking part of your daily routine

A main reason many people state for not walking or exercising regularly is lack of time. Make your walking program part of your daily routine the same as you fit your shower or favorite television program into your day. We tend to make time for what we want to make time for so make your walking a steadfast rule. Do it every day!

Be Flexible on Yourself

You know how important it is to have someone tell you they are proud of you. Tell yourself how proud you are of yourself after each session. If you are having a bad day, take a day off and don't beat yourself up over it. Acknowledge all that you've done and how great you've been about sticking with your schedule and track your progress so you can be proud.

Chapter 24 WHY WALKING IS SO IMPORTANT

Walking is a sport or pastime that more people are doing every day. There are so many reasons why walking is important beyond the very obvious: it's fun and great exercise. While the majority of the people that spend time walking do it for fitness, there are several reasons why we should all walk as much as possible.

A Healthier Environment

A large portion of the air pollution in the world comes from motor vehicles. According to the EPA, 55 percent of nitrogen oxide emissions and 80 percent of carbon monoxide in the United States is caused by transportation. Even though cars are being made better and cleaner, they still contribute to the worsening of our overall air quality. In addition, millions of barrels of oil, which is a non-renewable source of energy, are burnt every day by cars and trucks.

Less Roadway Congestion

We seldom stop to realize how short some of the trips we make in our cars really are. Approximately 40 percent of all trips made in the U.S. are under two miles, which is equal to a 30-minute walk. Many of the highways and streets are carrying more traffic than they were meant to handle, causing wasted energy, time, driver aggravation, pollution and overall congested roadways. Two pedestrians walking take up a lot less space than two people driving a car or truck.

Healthier Life for All

Walking is so good for our health. The benefits it can provide are extraordinary. Physical activity has always been recommended for good health, even if you can only manage 30 minutes a day, and walking is exceptionally good for many health benefits including:

- Reduced risk of heart disease, diabetes, stroke and other chronic diseases
- Provides you a stronger heart
- More positive mental outlook
- Lower health care costs
- Overall improved quality of life

Economics

Walking is free! It doesn't get much more economical than that. With the rising costs of fuel as well as wear and tear and regular maintenance on your vehicle, owning and operating a car is very expensive. In fact, transportation takes up a lot of your income each year. The more walking you can do the more money you will save that can be spent on other things. There are some situations where you can't walk but why not take advantage of the times when you can and get out there and walk. It just makes good sense.

Chapter 25. WALKING TIPS FOR GOOD FITNESS

Walking is a great form of exercise. Some of the many things that walking will do for you include strengthening your joints and muscles, helping to reduce cardiac disease, improving your outlook on life and leaving you with an overall sense of well-being. Although you may be walking for exercise for the many health benefits it provides, you are still going to want to get the most you can get out of your walking sessions. Whether you've been doing it for ages or are planning to start a regime of walking, here are a few tips to help you have a successful walking routine.

Use the Buddy System

Regardless of how much you may think you enjoy walking by yourself, everything is always more fun when you are with a friend. By finding a friend or buddy to walk with you, you are going to enjoy walking farther and longer because you will be enjoying the company you are with and not thinking of the distance. When we walk by ourselves, it is much easier to find an excuse to skip a day here and there. The maximum benefits will be achieved by walking only if it is done regularly. When you have a buddy to walk with you, you can both provide motivation that is often needed. Walking with a friend can also be much safer.

Mix it Up A Little

Walking is a lot of fun and is also great exercise but if you are walking the same distance on the same block and passing the same houses day after day, you are going to get bored rather quickly. If you make things a little different, your walk is going to be more interesting and pleasurable. If you are walking in your neighborhood, choose different blocks from time to time. If you have run out of streets, you may wish to go to the neighborhood park, by the beach or downtown to walk. You will be amazed at how much more enjoyable your walk is going to be when you are in a new area, giving yourself some new sightseeing options.

ABOUT THE AUTHOR

Hello, my name is Cindy Zahn. I graduated from the Institute for Integrative Nutrition as a certified health coach. I also have three certificates from the Doctor Sears Wellness Institute in Prime Time Health (Adults & Seniors), Lean Expectations (Pregnant Woman and new Moms) and Lean Start (Young Families).

In all of these programs I have been involved with, the main theme I kept hearing over and over again was the importance of diet and exercise. With your diet it is important to eat whole foods, that is food that is as close to natural as possible. Eating organic is best, but if you feel that it's not worth the extra cost, or maybe it is not available in your area, the non-organic will have to do. Exercise is equally important. When you exercise your blood is pumping faster through your blood vessels. This creates a thing called nitric oxide. Nitric oxide is a fundamental key in keeping your body healthy. Don't let anyone tell you that you can diet without exercise. It's like saying you can go swimming without water.

This book is the 4th in my "Don't just sit there" series of books. This series of books is all about getting out there and exercising. No excuses!

OTHER BOOKS BY CINDY ZAHN

Don't just sit there! How to get fit in 15 minutes a day.

Don't just sit there! The best way to learn yoga from home in 15 minutes a day for 21 days.

Don't just sit there! Start yoga for seniors now.

The healing power of food.

The souper diet.

Healing foods of the Bible.

The amazing apple: A wholefood wonder.

www.ingramcontent.com/pod-product-compliance
Lightning Source LLC
Chambersburg PA
CBHW07124328O526
45788CB00004B/1554